100% NATURAL CURE FOR BREAST CANCER AT ANY STAGE

UNDERSTANDING BREAST CANCER AND USING HERBAL OR ROOT TO CURE IT

U.S. ALEX

To the warriors, survivors, and thrivers; to those who have faced the challenges and uncertainties of breast cancer with unwavering strength and grace. Your resilience and courage have illuminated the path for all.

To the families and loved ones who provide unyielding support, comfort, and love to those affected by breast cancer. Your devotion is a powerful force.

To the healthcare professionals, researchers, and advocates who dedicate their lives to breast cancer care, research, and awareness. Your commitment is invaluable in the journey towards a breast cancer-free world.

To those who we've lost to breast cancer, your memory inspires our determination to find a cure and eliminate this disease.

And to every reader, seeking knowledge, understanding, and hope, may this book provide the information and inspiration you need on your journey through the world of breast cancer.

With profound respect for the breast cancer community and the countless lives touched by this disease.

CONTENTS

Title Page

Dedication

INTRODUCTION 1

What is Breast Cancer? 3

Risk Factors for Breast Cancer 4

Breast Cancer Statistics 6

ANATOMY OF THE BREAST 9

TYPES OF BREAST CANCER 15

CAUSES AND RISK FACTORS FOR BREAST CANCER 24

SYMPTOMS AND DIAGNOSIS OF BREAST CANCER 31

Diagnostic Checks for Breast Cancer 33

Breast Cancer Screening 35

STAGES OF BREAST CANCER 37

NATURAL REMEDIES FOR BREAST CANCER 40

HERBAL REMEDIES FOR BREAST CANCER 42

EMOTIONAL AND PSYCHOLOGICAL FACTORS OF BREAST CANCER 50

Coping With Cancer 52

BREAST CANCER RESEARCH AND FUTURE DIRECTIONS 58

CONCLUSION 62

About The Author 65

INTRODUCTION

Breast cancer is a form of cancer that starts in the milk ducts or lobules, which makes milk and usually affects the breast tissue.

This illness can occur in both males and females, but it's much more common among women. Depending on where the cancer cells are and what features they take on, breast cancer can be divided into diverse types such as invasive ductal carcinoma, DCIS, invasive lobular carcinoma, inflammatory breast cancer, and triple-negative breast cancer.

Symptoms that may imply this include a lump in the breast, changes in size/shape of the breast, nipple discharge, or changes in the skin of the breasts. That being said, some people don't show any symptoms. Risk factors associated with this illness include age, sex, family history of it, specific genetic mutations, early menstruation/late menopause onset, hormone therapy usage, and alcohol consumption. Doctors diagnose this through physical exams plus imaging & biopsy tests.

WHAT IS BREAST CANCER?

Breast cancer can be defined as a malignant disease that starts in the cells of the breast tissue. It is most frequently found in women but can occur in both sexes. If not correctly treated, it can spread to other fatal parts of the body. Despite being a grave condition, early diagnosis and treatment can meaningfully increase the chances of successful outcomes.

RISK FACTORS FOR BREAST CANCER

Many factors can raise the risk of developing breast cancer. Few risk factors are controllable, while others are not. Here are some common risk factors for breast cancer:

1.   As a person get old, their chances of developing breast cancer increase; most cases are diagnosed in women over 50 years.

2.   women are more likely to have breast cancer than men.

3.   Trait of breast cancer in a family lineage, such as in one's grandmother, mother, or sister can increase one's risk of contracting the disease.

4.   An inherited mutation in a gene can significantly raise your risk of getting breast cancer

5.   Estrogen and progesterone hormones for an extended period through

hormone replacement therapy or the use of contraceptives can significantly increase one's chance of growing breast cancer

6.   Excessive intake of alcohol daily has been linked to the risk of breast cancer.

7.   Obesity can elevate the likelihood of getting breast cancer, especially in women who have gone through menopause

8.   Exposed to radiation therapy during childhood may increase one's risk of developing breast cancer later in life.

9   Not engaging in physical activity regularly has been associated with a higher likelihood of developing breast cancer.

BREAST CANCER STATISTICS

Breast cancer is one of the most common cancers globally, millions of people are affected yearly. Here are some stats related to it:

• Breast cancer is the second most common type among women worldwide after lung cancer.

• and Over 685,000 women died from it in 2020, out of the estimated 2.3 million women who were diagnosed with it.

• In 2021 in the US, it's estimated that 281,000 women and 2,650 men will be diagnosed with it and 44,000 women and 500 men will die from it.

• In the US breast cancer is the most commonly diagnosed type among women excluding skin cancer.

- The risks of breast cancer are significant in elderly women, especially from 50 years and above.

- 5-10% of breast cancer cases are hereditary - caused by genetic mutations passed down through families.

- Mammography screenings and early detection can greatly increase the chances of successful treatment and well-being or recovery of breast cancer patients.

The Essence of Early Detection

1. Less harsh treatment: Cancer diagnoses early are usually less aggressive and require less intensive treatment, leading to fewer or no side effects and improved lifestyle for the patient.

2. Higher survival rate: Early detection significantly increases the five-year survival rate - nearly 100%, whereas when detected at an advanced stage, the chances for recovery are much lower.

3. More treatment options: If discovered sooner, there is a variety

of treatments such as less invasive surgeries, radiation therapy, and targeted drug therapies that can be used with greater success.

4. A sense of relief: Regular breast cancer screenings give you peace of mind knowing potential issues are being monitored proactively and addressed in due time.

5. Easier to manage: With early detection, treatment can start earlier making it simpler to manage and reducing recovery time

It is highly recommended that all women perform self-breast exams regularly, get screened as recommended by their physician, and report any changes or concerns immediately to their doctor for further evaluation.

ANATOMY OF THE BREAST

The breast is a glandular organ that is placed on the chest wall, consisting of multiple buildings that work together to produce and transport milk for the duration of lactation. Here are the important structures that make up the anatomy of the breast:

1. Areola: The areola is the darker location of skin surrounding the nipple.

2. Milk ducts: The milk ducts are thin tubes that carry milk from the lobules to the nipple.

3. Nipple: The nipple is the small, raised protrusion at the middle of the breast that releases milk during lactation.

4. Fatty tissue: The breast is surrounded by the aid of fatty tissue that presents assistance and protection for the glandular tissue.

5. Lobules: The lobules are small, spherical structures that produce milk in the course of lactation.

Structure of the Breast

The breast is composed of several sorts of tissue, inclusive of glandular tissue, connective tissue, adipose tissue, and blood vessels. Here is a brief overview of the structure of the breast:

1. Blood vessels and lymphatics: The breast is provided with the aid of a channel of blood vessels and lymphatic vessels, which elevate nutrients and oxygen to the breast tissue and do away with waste products.

2. Adipose tissue: Adipose tissue, also known as fatty tissue, surrounds the glandular tissue and provides cushioning and protection for the breast. The amount of adipose tissue in the breast varies from person to person and can be influenced by factors such as age, genetics, and overall body weight.

3. Areola and nipple: The areola is the darker pigmented place surrounding the nipple. The nipple is a raised, protruding shape that releases milk at some stage in lactation.

4. Nerves: The breast is innervated by using a network of nerves that provide sensation to the breast tissue.

5. Glandular tissue: The glandular tissue of the breast is accountable for producing milk. This tissue is made up of lobules, which are small, round constructions that incorporate milk-producing cells. These lobules are related to ducts, which lift milk to the nipple.

6. Connective tissue: The connective tissue of the breast includes ligaments and fibrous tissue that guide and structure the breast. Cooper's ligaments, which are skinny bands of tissue, provide help and assist keep the shape of the breast.

Functions of the Breast

The main feature of the breast is to produce milk to nourish a newborn. During pregnancy, hormones need breast tissue to develop and boost lactation. After childbirth, milk manufacturing starts and the baby can obtain integral nutrients from the mother's milk. Here are the principal functions of the breast:

1. Hormone production: The breast additionally produces hormones, such as estrogen and progesterone, which are essential for retaining reproductive fitness in women.

2. Lactation: Lactation is the procedure through which milk is released from the breast and made handy to the baby. This procedure is regulated by using hormones and can be influenced by the baby's feeding patterns.

3. Sensation: The breast carries several nerve endings that provide sensation to the breast tissue, making it an erogenous quarter for sexual stimulation.

4. Milk production: The breast produces milk to nourish a new child baby. Milk is produced via glandular tissue in the breast and

is transported via ducts to the nipple.

5. Body image: The appearance of the breasts can have a sizeable effect on a woman's self-image and body image.

Overall, the breast performs a vital function in reproductive health and the nourishment of a new child baby.

There are two principal sorts of breast tissue: glandular tissue and adipose tissue.

1. Adipose tissue: Adipose tissue, additionally recognized as fatty tissue, surrounds the glandular tissue and offers cushioning and safety for the breast. The amount of adipose tissue in the breast varies from character to man or woman and can be influenced with the aid of elements such as age, genetics, and average physique weight.

2. Glandular tissue: Glandular tissue is made up of lobules, which are small, spherical structures that produce milk at some stage in lactation. These lobules are linked to ducts, which carry milk to the nipple. Glandular tissue

is more every day in younger girls who have no longer gone thru menopause.

Both glandular tissue and adipose tissue can be current in distinct proportions in different women. The quantity of glandular tissue in the breast can affect a woman's capacity to breastfeed, whilst the amount of adipose tissue can affect the usual measurement and shape of the breast. Understanding the specific sorts of breast tissue is important for breast most cancers screening and diagnosis, as nicely as for breast reconstruction surgical operation after a mastectomy.

TYPES OF BREAST CANCER

There are numerous sorts of breast cancer, which are labeled based totally on the type of cells that are affected. Here are some of the most common kinds of breast cancer:

1.   Invasive ductal carcinoma (IDC)

2.   Ductal carcinoma in situ (DCIS)

3.   Invasive lobular carcinoma (ILC)

4.   Lobular carcinoma in situ (LCIS)

5.   Inflammatory breast most cancers (IBC)

6.   Triple-negative breast cancer

7.   HER2-positive breast cancer

1. Invasive Ductal Carcinoma (IDC)

Invasive ductal carcinoma (IDC) is the most common type of breast cancer, accounting for about 80% of all cases. IDC starts off evolving in the milk ducts of the breast, however, it can spread to the surrounding breast tissue and other parts of the body if left untreated. IDC is called "invasive" because most cancer cells have invaded the surrounding tissue.

Symptoms of IDC may additionally consist of a lump or thickening in the breast, changes in breast structure or size, nipple discharge, or an alternate appearance or texture of the breast skin. However, some girls with IDC can also now not experience any signs and symptoms at all.

The therapy for IDC generally involves an aggregate of surgery, radiation therapy, chemotherapy, and/or hormone therapy. The specific treatment design will depend on a range of factors, along with the dimension and place of the tumor, the stage of cancer, and the woman's average health.

The prognosis for IDC relies upon many factors, including the stage of cancer at the time of diagnosis, the woman's age and universal health, and how well most cancers respond to treatment. However, with early detection and fantastic treatment, many ladies with IDC are in a position to obtain long-term survival and an exact first-class life. It is vital for ladies to endure everyday breast cancer screening and to report any adjustments or abnormalities in their breasts to their healthcare provider.

2. Ductal Carcinoma in Situ (DCIS)

Ductal carcinoma in situ (DCIS) is a type of non-invasive breast most cancers that takes place in the milk ducts of the breast. DCIS is considered to be an early stage of most cancers and is commonly now not life-threatening, however, it does require therapy to forestall it from becoming invasive and spreading to different components of the breast or beyond.

DCIS is called "in situ" because most cancer cells have no longer spread beyond the ducts to invade the surrounding breast tissue. It is normally detected thru mammography, as it does not typically purpose any symptoms.

Treatment for DCIS commonly includes surgery to remove the cancerous cells, observed by way of radiation remedy to kill any remaining most cancers cells. In some cases, hormone therapy may also be encouraged to limit the chance of recurrence. If DCIS is detected early, the prognosis is typically very good, with a high likelihood of successful cure and long-term survival.

However, it is necessary to observe that some instances of DCIS can progress to invasive breast cancer if left untreated. Therefore, it is important for girls to bear ordinary breast cancer screening and to report any modifications or abnormalities in their breasts to their healthcare provider.

3. Invasive lobular carcinoma (ILC)

Invasive lobular carcinoma (ILC) is a kind of breast most cancers that starts in the lobules of the breast and can unfold to the surrounding tissue and different components of the body if left untreated. ILC money is owed for approximately 10-15% of all breast cancers.

Symptoms of ILC can also consist of a lump or thickening in the breast, adjustments in breast shape or size, nipple discharge, or an exchange in the appearance or texture of the breast skin. However, some girls with ILC can also not experience any signs and symptoms at all.

The remedy for ILC generally involves a mixture of surgery, radiation therapy, chemotherapy, and/or hormone therapy. The unique cure plan will rely on a variety of factors, along with the size and region of the tumor, the stage of cancer, and the woman's average health.

The prognosis for ILC depends on many factors, inclusive of the stage of most cancers at the time of diagnosis, the woman's age and ordinary health, and how properly most cancers respond to treatment. However, with early detection and gorgeous treatment, many girls with ILC are capable to obtain long-term survival and a truly pleasant life.

It is vital for women to undergo everyday breast cancer screening and to document any modifications or abnormalities in their breasts to their healthcare provider. Early detection and cure can radically enhance the prognosis for females with ILC.

4. Lobular Carcinoma in Situ (LCIS)

Lobular carcinoma in situ (LCIS) is a type of non-invasive breast cancer that happens in the lobules of the breast. LCIS is no longer regarded as a true cancer, but rather an indicator of an extended threat of creating invasive breast cancer in the future.

LCIS is commonly detected incidentally on a mammogram or biopsy, as it no longer commonly causes any symptoms. Women with LCIS have an improved chance of developing invasive breast cancer in both breasts, but the chance is higher in the breast the place LCIS was once diagnosed.

Treatment for LCIS normally involves shut monitoring with normal breast exams, mammograms, and/or MRI scans. Some females may also select to take medicines such as tamoxifen or aromatase inhibitors to reduce their danger of creating invasive breast cancer.

While LCIS is no longer real cancer, it is still vital for women in this situation to be vigilant about breast health and to endure everyday breast most cancers screening. This can help to observe any adjustments or abnormalities early when treatment is most effective.

Other less frequent types of breast cancer

In addition to invasive ductal carcinoma, invasive lobular carcinoma, ductal carcinoma in situ, and lobular carcinoma in situ, there are various other much less frequent sorts of breast cancer. These include:

1.   **Inflammatory Breast Cancers** (IBC): IBC is a rare and aggressive kind of breast cancer that bills for less than 5% of all breast cancer cases. IBC can purpose the breast to end up red, swollen, and heat to the touch, and it may purpose the skin to appear dimpled or pitted. Treatment for IBC typically includes chemotherapy, surgery, and radiation therapy.

2.   **Phyllodes Tumor**: Phyllodes tumors are uncommon breast tumors that advance in the connective tissue of the breast. Symptoms may also include a lump in the breast, breast pain, and a change in breast dimension or shape. Treatment for phyllodes tumors commonly includes surgery, and in some cases, radiation therapy.

3.   **Angiosarcoma**: Angiosarcoma is a rare type of breast most cancers that develops in the blood vessels or lymph vessels of the breast. Symptoms may also include a lump in the breast, breast pain, and swelling or redness of the breast. Treatment for angiosarcoma typically entails surgery, chemotherapy, and/or

radiation therapy.

4.   **Paget's Disorder of The Nipple**: Paget's disease of the nipple is a rare structure of the breast most cancers that impacts the skin of the nipple and the areola. Symptoms may also encompass itching, redness, flaking, or crusting of the nipple and a lump or thickening in the breast. Treatment for Paget's disease of the nipple commonly involves surgical procedures and radiation therapy.

CAUSES AND RISK FACTORS

FOR BREAST CANCER

1   Genetic factor

Genetic factors can play a major role in the development of breast cancer. Inherited gene mutations, such as BRCA1 and BRCA2, are the most standard genetic risk factors for breast cancer. Women who inherit a mutated replica of either of these genes have an appreciably extended chance of creating breast cancer, as nicely as an expanded hazard of developing ovarian cancer.

Other less frequent inherited gene mutations, such as TP53, PALB2, and CHEK2, are also related to an accelerated threat of breast cancer.

It's important to know that inherited gene mutations account for a small proportion of breast cancer cases (about 5-10%), and most instances of breast cancers are not prompted with the aid of inherited gene mutations.

In addition to inherited gene mutations, somatic mutations can additionally play a function in the development of breast cancer. These somatic mutations can be triggered by environmental elements (such as exposure to radiation or chemicals) or other factors that injure DNA, such as normal growing old processes.

2. **Hormonal elements**

Hormonal factors can also play a role in the development of breast cancer. Estrogen and progesterone, two hormones produced by way of the ovaries, can stimulate the increase of breast cells. Exposure to these hormones over a long period increases the chance of developing breast cancer.

Some factors that can increase a woman's exposure to estrogen and progesterone include:

i. Late onset of menopause: Women who go through menopause later in life (after age 55) have a longer exposure to estrogen and progesterone, which can enlarge their chance of developing breast cancer.

ii. Early onset of menstruation: Women who begin menstruating at a younger age (before age 12) are exposed to greater menstrual cycles over their lifetime, which can make bigger their hazard of creating breast cancer.

iii. Hormone replacement remedy (HRT): Women who use hormone replacement therapy (HRT) to manipulate menopause signs (such as hot flashes) are exposed to additional estrogen and progesterone, which can amplify their hazard of developing breast cancer.

iv. Oral contraceptives: Some researchers have suggested that ladies who use oral contraceptives (birth control pills) might also have a slightly expanded risk of developing breast cancer, especially if they use them for a lengthy period.

v.   Pregnancy and breastfeeding: Women who have children and breastfeed them have a lower threat of developing breast cancer, perchance because being pregnant and breastfeeding limit a woman's publicity to estrogen and progesterone.

It's essential to observe that whilst hormonal elements can extend a woman's chance of growing breast cancer, no longer all females who are uncovered to high levels of estrogen and progesterone will strengthen the disease. Other factors, such as genetics and environmental factors, additionally play a role.

3. Lifestyle factors

A certain way of lifestyle has additionally been linked to an accelerated threat of breast cancer. These include:

i.   Physical inactivity: Women who are now not physically active have a higher danger of developing breast most cancers in contrast to women who engage in ordinary physical activity.

ii.   Obesity: Women who are overweight or chubby have a greater chance of developing breast cancer, particularly after menopause.

iii.   Alcohol consumption: Women who consume alcohol commonly have a higher chance of developing breast cancers in contrast to women who do not drink alcohol.

iv.   Smoking: Although smoking has not been directly linked to breast cancer, it can make bigger the threat of other cancers, such as lung cancer, and can additionally have terrible results on universal health.

v.   Diet: There is some evidence to endorse that a diet excessive in saturated fats and low in fruits and vegetables can also extend the chance of breast cancer.

It's vital to observe that making lifestyle changes, such as exercising regularly, preserving a healthy weight, and limiting alcohol consumption, can assist to decrease a woman's risk of growing breast cancer.

4. Environmental factors

Environmental elements may additionally also contribute to the improvement of breast cancer. These elements can include:

i. Radiation exposure: Exposure to excessive tiers of radiation, such as from medical imaging assessments or radiation therapy, can expand the hazard of creating breast cancer.

ii. Chemical exposure: Exposure to sure chemicals, such as those discovered in some pesticides, plastics, and industrial products, can also expand the chance of growing breast cancer.

iii. Air pollution: Exposure to air pollution, especially in urban areas, has been linked to an elevated chance of breast cancer.

iv. Night shift work: Women who work night time shifts may have an elevated danger of growing breast cancer, possibly due to disruptions in the body's circadian rhythm.

v. Geographical location: Studies have proven that women who stay in certain geographical areas, such as those with excessive ranges of industrial pollution or publicity to agricultural chemicals, may additionally have a greater hazard of growing breast cancer.

It's important to be aware that whilst environmental factors can also play a function in the development of breast cancer, their exact contribution is nonetheless being studied.

SYMPTOMS AND DIAGNOSIS

OF BREAST CANCER

Symptoms of breast cancer may additionally include:

A. A lump or thickening in the breast or underarm area
B. Changes in the size or shape of the breast
C. Nipple discharge or nipple turning inward (inverted nipple)
D. Skin dimpling or puckering
E. Redness, scaling, or swelling of the breast or nipple
F. Breast pain that is new or persistent

However, it is essential to notice that no longer all breast lumps or changes are cancerous. Many benign (non-cancerous) breast conditions can have similar symptoms, such as **fibroadenomas or cysts.**

If a girl notices any difference in her breasts, she should speak to her doctor. The healthcare provider may additionally function a body examination and order imaging tests, such as a mammogram or ultrasound, to decide the reason for the changes.

If breast cancer is noticed, a biopsy may additionally be carried out. A biopsy includes getting a sample of tissue from the breast and analyzing it under a microscope to look for most cancer cells. In some cases, breast cancer may additionally be detected via activities screening tests, such as mammograms. Early detection and therapy of breast cancers can enlarge the probability of a profitable cure. It's essential for women to operate breast self-exams oftentimes and to have normal breast tests via a healthcare provider.

DIAGNOSTIC CHECKS FOR

BREAST CANCER

Diagnostic tests for breast cancers are mostly used to verify an analysis of breast cancers after a suspicious area has been discovered at some stage in a screening check or bodily exam. These checks might also include:

1. Biopsy: A biopsy is a method in which a small sample of tissue is taken from the breast and examined underneath a microscope to search for cancer cells. There are extraordinary kinds of biopsies, such as core needle biopsy, surgical biopsy, and nice needle aspiration.

2. Imaging tests: Imaging tests, such as ultrasound, mammograms, and magnetic resonance imaging (MRI), can assist furnish extra information about the suspicious vicinity in the breast. These exams can help determine the dimension and place of the abnormality and whether it has unfolded to other areas of the breast or nearby lymph nodes.

3. Breast ductal lavage: This is a newer check that includes washing a small amount of fluid from the milk ducts and examining it below a microscope to look for atypical cells.

4. Blood tests: Blood assessments are not used to diagnose breast cancer, but they may additionally be used to take a look at particular proteins, such as CA-15-3 or CA 27.29, which can be improved in people with breast cancer. These checks are often used to screen the development of treatment.

BREAST CANCER SCREENING

Breast cancer screening includes the use of checks or exams to realize breast cancer earlier than any signs are present. The goal of screening is to identify breast cancer at an early stage when it's most treatable. There are countless types of breast cancer screening tests, including:

1. Mammogram: A mammogram is when an X-ray is carried out on the breast. It's the most frequent screening check for breast cancer nowadays. During a mammogram, the breast is compressed between two plates and X-ray pictures are taken from one-of-a-kind angles.
2. Breast self-exam: A breast self-exam includes a patient inspecting her breasts for any lumps or changes. While breast self-exams are no longer an alternative to regular mammograms or medical breast exams, they can assist girls to end up acquainted with how their breasts normally seem to be any sense and can assist discover modifications early
3. Clinical breast exam: A clinical breast exam is a bodily

examination of the breast performed by a healthcare provider. The provider will seem to feel for any lumps or other abnormalities in the breast.

4. Breast MRI: A breast MRI uses magnetic fields and radio waves to create certain photographs of the breast. It may also be endorsed for women who have a greater threat of breast cancer, such as those with a strong family history of the disease.

STAGES OF BREAST CANCER

Breast cancer is classified into stages based on the size of the tumor, whether or not it has unfolded to nearby lymph nodes or other components of the body, and different factors. The levels of breast most cancers are:

I.   Stage 0: Also known as ductal carcinoma in situ (DCIS), this is an early stage of breast cancer where unusual cells are found in the milk ducts of the breast yet to spread beyond the ducts.

II.   Stage I: This is an early stage of invasive breast cancer; at this stage, the tumor is small (less than two centimeters) and has yet to unfold to the lymph nodes or different parts of the body.

III.   Stage II: This stage can be divided into two sub-stages:

Stage IIA: The tumor is nonetheless small (less than 2 centimeters) however has unfolded to the

axillary lymph nodes (located in the armpit) or the

tumor is large (between 2-5 centimeters)

however, has not yet spread to the lymph nodes.

Stage IIB: The tumor is a bit large (between 2-5 centimeters) and has unfolded to the axillary

lymph nodes or the tumor is large than 5 centimeters but has not unfolded to the lymph nodes.

IV.   Stage III: This stage is divided into three sub-stages:

Stage IIIA: The tumor may also be any size and has spread to the axillary lymph nodes, which

are now sticking collectively or to surrounding tissues, or the tumor is large than 5 centimeters

and has unfolded to the axillary lymph nodes.

Stage IIIB: Most cancers have unfolded to the skin,

chest wall, or lymph nodes close to the

breastbone, and may or may additionally no longer have spread to the axillary lymph nodes.

Stage IIIC: The cancer has spread to lymph nodes above or beneath the collarbone, and may

also, or may additionally not have unfolded to the axillary lymph nodes.

V.   Stage IV: Also referred to as metastatic breast cancer, this is the most superior stage of breast cancer the place the cancer has spread to other components of the body, such as the bones, liver, lungs, or brain.

The stage of breast most cancers helps healthcare companies decide the most excellent therapy format for an individual.

NATURAL REMEDIES FOR

BREAST CANCER

The treatment of breast cancer strictly depends on quite a few elements such as the stage of cancer, kind of breast cancer, hormone receptor status, HER2 status, and the person's universal health. The most common redress for breast cancers are:

1. Radiation therapy: Radiation remedy makes use of high-energy radiation to kill most cancer cells and cut back tumors. It is frequently used after surgery to kill any closing cancer cells and decrease the risk of recurrence.
2. Surgery: Surgery is quite often a remedy for breast cancer, and the aim is to take away the cancerous tumor and some of the surrounding tissue. Types of surgical operation for breast cancer include lumpectomy (removal of the tumor and a small amount of surrounding tissue), mastectomy (removal of the whole breast), and lymph node surgery (removal of some or all of the lymph nodes underneath the arm).
3. Chemotherapy: Chemotherapy makes use of drugs to terminate most cancer cells throughout the body part. It can also be prescribed earlier than or after surgery,

depending on the stage of cancer.

4. Targeted therapy: Targeted remedy uses pills with unique proteins on cancer cells. For example, HER2-positive breast cancers can be dealt with with focused therapy drugs that target the HER2 protein.

5. Hormone therapy: Hormone remedy is used to treat breast cancers that are hormone receptor-positive. It blocks the consequences of estrogen on breast most cancers cells and may be given for quite a few years.

HERBAL REMEDIES FOR

BREAST CANCER

Echinacea

Echinacea belongs to the family Asteraceae. It is an uninhabited aromatic plant that cultivates mainly in the Great Plains and eastern regions of North America and is also produced in Europe. For herbal remedies three types of species are most commonly found, named as Echinacea purpurea, Echinacea angustifolia, and Echinacea pallida. But for research and treatment, E. purpurea is most commonly used

Flavonoids act as an immune stimulant, they are present in Echinacea. It was supported by Winston et al., and flavonoids promote the lymphocyte's activity that increases the phagocytosis by macrophages and the action of natural killer cells and prompting interferon assembly, and it has also reduced the harmful consequence of radiotherapy and chemotherapy. It also helps the patients in prolonging the survival time with the progressive stage of cancer.

Garlic

Garlic (Allium sativum), for hundreds of years, has been used for treating many illnesses. It involves a hundred or more hundred therapeutically useful secondary metabolites, for example, alliin, alliinase, and allicin. Alliin, an amino acid, is present in garlic oil that is transformed into allicin after its rhizomes are crumpled. An originator of Sulfur comprising compound is allicin, which is responsible for odor and its therapeutic properties. Garlic oil contains another Sulfur holding substance, Ajoene. Ajoene delays cancer production while selenium is an antioxidant. Bioflavonoids, cyanidin, and quercetin are also found in garlic with antioxidant properties.

Turmeric

The scientific name of turmeric is Curcuma longa. Turmeric gives a dark yellow color to food. Curcumin, the active ingredient of turmeric, is present in its rhizome and rootstock. Curcumin is known to have anti-cancerous activity due to its phenolic substances. Propagation of lung, breast, skin, and stomach cancer is limited by turmeric.

It has also anti-inflammatory action in humans. Curcumin has been revealed to have inhibitory action in all phases of cancer growth which are initiation, promotion, and propagation. Nitrosamine production is inhibited by turmeric; it results in increased natural antioxidant action in the body. The amount of glutathione and other non-protein sulphydryl is increased by curcumin, and they act directly on different enzymes

Burdock

Scientific name of Burdock is Arctium lappa. Its root is found and used in Europe and Asia. There are many therapeutic uses of burdock in herbal remedies. Its root has a gummy texture and sweet taste. In old times burdock was useful in arthritis, tonsillitis, and measles, but nowadays it has been found that burdock has antitumor activity. It contains some active ingredients that alter the changes in oncogenes. Burdock has been utilized in the treatment of breast tumors, ovaries, bladder, malignant melanoma, lymphoma, and pancreatic cells. It relieves the pain, lessens the tumor size, and enhances the survival phase. To withstand the fast propagation and division of cells, a huge amount of nutrients is required during cancer.

Carotenoids

An active compound known as "carotenoids" is possessed by green, herbs with leaves, and rose hips. These aromatic plants are used as dyeing agents for example saffron, annatto, and paprika. Consumption of vegetables and fruits has been linked with less expansion of different forms of tumors. Intake of carotenoids through diet also decreases the occurrence of tumors.

Green tea

Scientifically green tea is known as Camellia sinensis. Anticancer activity is attributed to polyphenolic compounds. Epigallocatechin (EGGG), a polyphenol is present in small amounts in C. sinensis. Researchers have revealed that green tea possesses antitumor and anti-mutagenic activity. Cells are protected by EGGG from DNA damage produced by oxygen-reactive species Studies on animal were performed resulted that green tea polyphenols restricts the cancer cell division and stimulate the necrosis and apoptosis of tumor cells. While the function of the immune system is stimulated by tea catechins, they also inhibit metastases and angiogenesis in tumor cells.

Ginseng

Scientific name of ginseng is Panax ginseng. It is a lasting plant mainly grown in China, Korea, Japan, and Russia. Part used of this plant is dried root. It has many therapeutic uses including cancer. Active substances of ginseng have been shown that reduces or block the development of tumor necrosis factor in the skin of a mouse, block the propagation and metastases of cancerous cells, and stimulate cell differentiation and level of interferon.

Black cohosh

Scientific name of black cohosh is Cimicifuga recemosa. It is a shrub, found in the eastern forests of North America. Patients of breast cancer most commonly used Black cohosh during radiotherapy and chemotherapy. It has been used by Native Americans for many centuries for the treatment of menopausal signs, pre-menstrual discomfort, and dysmenorrhea.

Flax seed

Flax plant has small brown and golden hard-coated seeds. These small seeds contain all active components. Flax seeds are a rich source of dietary fiber, omega-3 fat, and lignans. Estrogenic activity is present in flax seeds due to the metabolism of lignans to enterodiol and enterolactone, and metabolism occurs in the digestive tract. As compared to soy products, flax seeds have more potent phytoestrogens, while intake of flax seeds causes a huge change in the elimination of 2-hydoxyesterone than soy protein

Vitamin D

Vitamin D is produced by sun exposure to the skin. A large amount of vitamin D is produced by simple contact of hands, arms, and face in summer. Even standing in the sunshine on the beach until the pinkness of the skin is equal to a 20,000 IU oral dose of vitamin D2. A minimal amount of vitamin required by our body is 1000 IU/day, to maintain the sufficient level.

EMOTIONAL AND PSYCHOLOGICAL

FACTORS OF BREAST CANCER

Breast cancer can have a huge emotional and psychological impact on a person. Some common emotional and psychological elements of breast cancer include:

1. Anxiety
2. Depression
3. Fear
4. Body photograph concerns.
5. Relationship and intimacy issues
6. Financial concerns

It's paramount to tackle the emotional and psychological elements of breast cancer alongside clinical treatment. Talking to an intellectual health expert or becoming a member of a support team can be useful in coping with these challenges.

It's additionally important to connect with loved ones and communicate how you are feeling and prioritize self-care during the breast cancer journey.

COPING WITH CANCER

Breast cancer can be overwhelming and emotional, and it can be hard to recognize how to cope. Here are some suggestions for coping with breast cancer:

1. Build an assist network: Reach out to friends, and family, and assist businesses for emotional support. Consider becoming a member of a team of people with breast cancer to connect with others who are going through comparable experiences.
2. Educate yourself: Learn as much as you can about breast cancer. This can help you experience more in managing and getting better prepared.
3. Take care of your health: Eat a healthy diet, get regular exercise, and observe your doctors' pointers for managing the side effects of treatment.
4. Practice stress-reducing techniques: Consider meditation, yoga, or different stress-reducing strategies to help manipulate the emotional effect of breast cancer.
5. Stay positive: Try to center your attention on the positivity in your life, and look for opportunities to enjoy pleasure and which means even while dealing with breast cancer.
6. Consider speaking to a mental fitness professional: It's common to feel anxious or depressed after a breast

cancer diagnosis, and speaking to a mental fitness expert can assist you cope with these feelings.

Remember, coping with breast cancer is a journey, and it is vital to take care of your body. Reach out for guidance when you need it, and be firm with yourself as you navigate this challenging experience.

Support For Breast Cancers Patients and Caregivers

Breast cancer can be challenging for each patient and their caregivers. Each needs to have access to aid and resources during the breast cancer journey. Here are some types of aid that might also be available:

Counseling or therapy: Talking to a mental health professional can help cope with the emotional and psychological factors of breast cancer. Many healthcare companies offer counseling offerings or can supply referrals to intellectual health professionals.

Support groups: Support groups for humans with breast cancer can provide a sense of community and connection with others who recognize what you're going through. Many support businesses are accessible online, making it easier to join with others from the alleviation of your very own home.

Educational resources: Educational resources, such as books, online resources, or classes, can grant facts on breast cancer treatment, side effects, and coping strategies.

Financial assistance: Breast most cancers remedy can be expensive, and monetary assistance packages may additionally be accessible to help cover the price of treatment.

Peer mentoring programs: Peer mentoring packages suit breast most cancers patients with survivors who can supply emotional help and practice based on their very own experiences.

Caregiver support: Caregivers may additionally also need assistance and resources to cope with the challenges of caring for anyone with breast cancer. Support groups, counseling, and academic assets can be useful for caregivers as well.

It's important to understand that assistance appears specific for everyone, and it is okay to are searching for out the kind of support that works pleasant for you. Your healthcare provider can grant suggestions on reachable resources, and companies such as the American Cancer Society and Susan G. Komen also provide a range of aid offerings for breast cancer sufferers and caregivers.

Lifestyle Changes to Enhance Fine of Life

Lifestyle changes can be an essential phase of enhancing the pleasant life for breast most cancers patients and survivors. Here are some way-of-life adjustments that may be helpful:

Nutrition: A healthy weight loss plan can assist increase strength ranges and assist universal health. Focus on a food regimen wealthy in fruits, vegetables, total grains, lean protein, and healthy fats.

Stress management: Managing stress can help enhance mood and limit anxiety. Techniques such as deep breathing, meditation, or yoga can be helpful.

Exercise: Regular exercising can improve mood, energy levels, and ordinary quality of life. It can also assist reduce the hazard of recurrence for breast cancer survivors. Aim for at least 150 minutes of reasonable workouts or 75 minutes of energetic exercise per week.

Sleep: Getting ample sleep is essential for ordinary fitness and well-being. Aim for 7-8 hours of sleep per night, and discuss with your healthcare company if you're having a hassle sleeping.

Limiting alcohol intake: Excessive alcohol consumption can make bigger the threat of breast cancer recurrence. Limit alcohol consumption to no more than one drink per day.

Smoking cessation: Quitting smoking can enhance standard fitness and minimize the danger of most cancers' recurrence. Talk to your healthcare issuer for assets and help to quit smoking.

BREAST CANCER RESEARCH

AND FUTURE DIRECTIONS

Breast cancer research is ongoing, and there are many areas at the center of attention for future directions. Here are some examples of cutting-edge and future lookup instructions in breast cancer:

1. Personalized medicine: Researchers are working to develop remedies that are tailor-made to individual sufferers primarily based on their unique genetic make-up and tumor characteristics.

2. Precision screening: Researchers are working to strengthen greater accurate and particular screening strategies for breast cancer, such as the use of genetic testing to perceive girls who are at excessive hazard for breast cancer.

3. Immunotherapy: Immunotherapy is a kind of cancer cure that uses the body's immune device to fight most cancer cells. Researchers are exploring the attainable of immunotherapy for breast cancer treatment.

4. Early detection: Early detection of breast cancer is fundamental for successful treatment. Researchers are working to increase new techniques for detecting breast cancer at a previous stage, such as via the use of imaging

applied sciences or blood tests.

5. Understanding most cancers biology: Researchers are working to better recognize the biology of breast cancer, including the genetic and molecular mechanisms that power the disease.

6. Survivorship: Researchers are working to enhance the first-class of lifestyles for breast most cancers survivors, via developing interventions to control long-term facet consequences of treatment, such as fatigue or pain.

Contemporary Findings on Breast Cancer

Breast most cancers research is a dynamic field, and discoveries are constantly being made. Here are some examples of cutting-edge lookup on breast cancer:

Genomic testing: Genomic testing is a kind of checking out that appears at the genes in a person's tumor to become aware of precise mutations or alterations that could be centered using treatment. Researchers are working to improve more particular genomic checking out methods for breast cancer, which should lead to greater positive and personalized remedy approaches.

Immunotherapy: Immunotherapy is a kind of most cancers cure that makes use of the body's immune system to combat most cancer cells. Researchers are presently exploring the plausibility of immunotherapy for breast most cancers treatment, along with the use of checkpoint inhibitors and CAR T-cell therapy.

Liquid biopsies: Liquid biopsies are a type of blood take a look at that can discover cancer cells or DNA fragments in the blood. Researchers are exploring the plausibility of liquid biopsies for detecting breast cancers before the stage and for monitoring cure response.

Combination therapies: Combination remedies involve the use of more than one drug or treatment modalities in the mixture to improve cure effectiveness. Researchers are exploring one-of-a-kind mixtures of chemotherapy, centered therapy, and immunotherapy for breast cancer treatment.

Breast cancer prevention: Researchers are working to develop new strategies for breast most cancers prevention, which includes the use of chemoprevention drugs, way-of-life modifications, and hazard-reduction surgery.

Survivorship: Researchers are working to enhance the best of life for breast most cancers survivors, by way of growing interventions to manage long-term facet effects of treatment, such as fatigue or pain.

Overall, breast most cancers research is centered on improving our understanding of the disease, developing more effective treatments, and improving results for patients.

CONCLUSION

Breast cancer is a complex disorder that affects millions of human beings worldwide. Although significant progress has been made in understanding the disease, there is still a lot to be learned. Early detection is necessary for successful treatment, and ladies are educated to carry out regular breast self-exams and to seek medical attention if they are aware of any adjustments in their breasts. Treatment options for breast cancer include chemotherapy, surgery, radiation therapy, and hormone therapy, among others, and the choice of therapy will depend on a variety of factors, which include the patient's character fitness status, and the stage of the disease.

The Significance of Breast Cancer Awareness

Breast cancer awareness helps ladies understand their risk factors for breast cancer and take steps to limit their risk, such as preserving a wholesome lifestyle and present process everyday screening. Early detection is key to profitable treatment, and girls who are aware of the signs and symptoms of breast most cancers are greater probable to seek scientific attention if they notice any changes in their breasts.

Secondly, breast cancer awareness helps limit the stigma surrounding the disease. Many females who are known for breast cancer feel ashamed or embarrassed, however, cognizance campaigns help to normalize the disease and inspire open discussions about it. This, in turn, can assist minimize emotions of isolation and enhance the pleasantness of existence for women residing with breast cancer.

Finally, breast cancer awareness helps raise funds to look up to the disease. Research is essential for growing new treatments and sooner or later discovering a cure for breast cancer. Awareness campaigns can help generate public interest and help research efforts, which can finally save lives.

In conclusion, breast cancer awareness is imperative for decreasing the burden of breast cancer on persons and society as a whole. By merchandising awareness, we can motivate females to take steps to limit their risk, minimize stigma and isolation, and generate assistance for research into this essential disease.

ABOUT THE AUTHOR

U.s. Alex

Dr. U.S.ALEX is a highly respected researcher with over two decades of experience in the field of medicine. I have made significant contributions to the medical field through her clinical work, research, and her role in mentoring the next generation of medical professionals. I have published numerous articles in reputable medical journals and have been at the forefront of groundbreaking research in areas such as cardiovascular medicine and preventive healthcare.

My motivation as an author of medical books is to bridge the gap between medical knowledge and patient understanding. She is deeply committed to making complex medical concepts accessible to the general public and to healthcare professionals seeking to expand their knowledge.

This book covers a wide range of medical topics, from comprehensive guides on specific medical conditions and their treatments to books focusing on wellness, nutrition, and lifestyle choices for maintaining optimal health. My works provide valuable insights for patients, caregivers, and healthcare practitioners alike.

As a medical author, my work serves as a valuable resource for those seeking to better understand medical conditions, treatment options, and the importance of maintaining good health. Her dedication to improving healthcare literacy and her contributions to medical literature have positively impacted countless lives.